CUM - Pocket Guide On How To Make Her Come & Orgasm

The Dark Arts Of Female Arousal, Orgasmic Sex Positions To Make Her Come & Last Longer In Bed!

by Alex Xavier

ISBN-13: 978-1976318146
ISBN-10: 1976318149

A Gentlemen's Pocket Guide To Sex & Orgasm

Dark Arts Of Female Arousal - How To Make Her Come Hard & Orgasmic Sex Positions That Keep Her Coming Back For More!

own research before making any purchase online.

Adherence to all applicable laws and regulations, including international, federal, state, and local governing professional licensing, business practices, advertising, and all other aspects of doing business in the US, Canada, Australia or any other jurisdiction is the sole responsibility of the reader or purchaser.

Neither the author nor the publisher assumes any responsibility or liability whatsoever on the behalf of the purchaser or reader of these materials. Any perceived slight of any individual or organization is purely unintentional.

Table of Contents

Free Gift

**Download "10 Tools For Stronger Erections" At:
http://bit.ly/10strongerection**

So you know how to make her come using orgasmic sex positions but do you want to get stronger erections?

Download this check list and get the 10 tools to help you with stronger erections so that you can last longer in bed.

**Download "10 Tools For Stronger Erections" At:
http://bit.ly/10strongerection**

Introduction

Ever wanted to learn the dark secrets of female arousal, how to make her come hard and experience intense orgasms?

Do you want to be the best lover she's ever had in bed and make her come back to you begging for more?

Hey, I'm Alex and no… I'm not a doctor, sex coach or some so called "expert". I'm an average guy who happens to have a fair deal of experience in dating and sleeping with beautiful women.

I wrote this pocket guide for men because my friends were constantly asking me for advice on "how they could last longer in bed" and how to give their ladies orgasms.

This book outlines the dark secret arts of female arousal and orgasmic sex positions based on REAL LIFE experiences with women *(not some magazine fluff)*.

A word of warning: This book is pretty "X-rated".

I'm going to be using words like "fuck", "pussy", "clit" etc and say things as they are… so if you're going to be offended - then STOP reading right now.

Also, this book is deliberately short for a reason.

I've seen so many BS filler books out there and it pisses me off badly. I want you to

SUCCEED and this book only provides you with the methods that **work**.

Less is more.

Yes, I've read the 64 kuma sutra positions and whilst they are good, who the heck has time to remember all those positions?

I even read a medical text book on the female anatomy to make sure that the information provided in this book is correct and not from my imagination.

At the end of the day, there really are a just a handful of secrets and sexual positions that you need to know to get her to scream and come hard.

Enough rambling… let's begin.

How It All Began…

Before I divulge the dark arts of female arousal and how to make her come hard… let me give you a background to how I came up with these techniques.

It all started in college when I took an interest in studying the human anatomy since my girlfriend at the time was in med school. As I began telling my friends how fascinating the human body was…

The one question that got asked ALOT by the boys was "how can I be REALLY great in bed - how can I be so good that chicks just want to "cum" back for more?"

Pardon the pun ;)

They seemed to think that with my *basic* knowledge of anatomy I would be able to give them some secret technique or formula that would give them the ability to give any woman intense, multiple orgasms.

The truth was that despite reading the medical text book studies, I didn't have the answer to these important questions. What wasn't a mystery to me, of course, was why they wanted to know how to do this.

It goes without saying that if you can give a woman incredible toe curling orgasms, then obviously - you've got power as a man.

The truth is that most guys are pretty hopeless when it comes to pleasing a woman in bed (no offense fellas... that's just what most women tell me).

This means that a rare opportunity exists for the man who really knows how to please a woman in bed. I'm not just talking about a man who can make a woman think "oh that was great sex"....

I'm talking about a man who can do things to a woman to

make her think "OMG, I never
knew my body could feel like
that, who is this freak? I have
to find a way to keep him
around me".

Once a woman has had such
a man she will never want to
give him up. He will take up a
special place in her mind and
she will always want to go
back for "more".

Do You Want To Become That Man?

Sure you do. If not then you are either gay, an old man who doesn't have sex anymore or maybe even a gay old man.

And by the way, there is nothing wrong with being gay or old, I'm just saying that you are if you don't want to learn these techniques. No offense meant okay… gay old dudes?

So to get back to where I was before, I got asked these questions about how to "get a woman off" and make "her come hard" so often and by so many different guys that eventually i figured that it was up to me *(with my superior medical knowledge about the female anatomy lol)* to find out the answers.

To accomplish this MASSIVE task, it took me several years of intense "study" in the field.

Firstly, I started by going over the painstaking detail of all the anatomy books I could find specifically those that focused on the female anatomy.

There was all these complex nerve endings, tendons, ligaments and potentially hidden erogenous zones that you don't learn in everyday life.

What I found was that anatomy texts books (whilst fascinating) couldn't give a hoot about which part of a

woman's sexual organs gave
her the most pleasure or what
area could be stimulated to
make her reach climax.

You see, these text books
were written purely for
scientific and medically
purposes only and were not
intended for a young male
who was trying to gather
knowledge to become the
world's greatest lover.

After gathering all the
anatomical and physiological
knowledge that I could, I

decided to go and speak to sex therapists to see if they could help me with the knowledge that I was looking for.

To my great surprise, not many sex therapist could actually give me the "dirt" I was looking for to give a woman mind blowing sex.

Or if they did know how, they sure as hell were not telling me.

Then one day, after months
and months of "research" just
as I was just about to give up
and put this project into the
"too hard basket", I was struck
by a bolt of lightning…
actually struck by a gorgeous
woman met through a mutual
friend.

This particular "friend" is what
we call a high-class escort.
She is trained in the art of
pleasing men, is incredibly
attractive and drips sex
appeal but that is another
matter.

As we were chatting, the topic of female orgasms came up and I told her about my recent failure to find out how to become a woman's greatest lover and make her reach multiple intense orgasms.

She laughed out loud when I told her how I had spoken to numerous sex therapists and proceeded to give me a suggestion that totally turned my life around.

Although at the time I had no idea how much of an impact it would make on me and of the many women I have pleasured since then and on other men that I have taught these techniques to.

She told me that if I wanted to know how to please a woman, then I needed to ask the women who were most experienced in that area - which was women like herself.

She told me quite openly that she has slept with hundreds

of men and has experienced
all sorts of men of different
sizes shapes and races with
an abundance of different
techniques and sexual styles
between them.

My jaw dropped... I then
asked her, "Of the hundreds
of men you have had sex
with, how many of them
actually gave you the sort of
mind boggling orgasms that
would keep you coming back
for more and more?"

She looked at me and thought
for a moment and said -
"Maybe 10.". I said "only 10?"
And she said, "yep."

I have to say that with what I
had heard already about most
men not knowing what to do
with a woman sexually *(even
though they think they do)* I
was expecting a low number,
but this was even far lower
than what I was expecting.

So I was all ears from this
point on and eagerly taking
notes from this high-class

escort *(let's refer to her as Alicia)* but there was a catch. She was only willing to give me everything she knew.... for a fee (which by the way was not small).

I arranged for Alicia and 5 of her most trusted friends in the same industry to sit down with me and divulge all the dirty tricks they knew.

There were many different techniques and tips discussed but at the end of the day, there were a few clear winners. Things that stood out far above the rest and things that all men must know if they want to keep their woman satisfied.

Some of these tips were quite general and some were quite specific but at the end of the day if you can master them then you will be living a life of endless sexual opportunities...

Which is not exactly a bad thing... and you can trust me on that one.

So here they are, in
sequential order, the dark arts
of female arousal that will
make her beg for more and
for your broader education
and development.

With all of the time and effort
that went into getting this
information, I should really be
charging a small fortune for
this information but I want to
give back to the community….

Just don't share these secrets
with too many guys or we will

lose our competitive
advantage...

CHAPTER ONE

Dark Secret Arts of Female Arousal & Orgasm

Dark Secret Number 1: Women Have Dirty Minds too

Yes, you heard it. I know I was surprised too, but apparently even the sweetest most innocent woman conjures up fantasies in her own head that would make most men blush.

Bullshit? Yes I thought so too when I heard it for the first time, but since being told this by "the panel" I have asked many of my girlfriends and casual sexual partners the same thing and initially I am met by the same response.

"Oh shut up, is that all you think about," or *"OMG, we are not like you okay"* or *"God can you guys just get over that weird kinky shit already".*

All these responses are programmed into woman to throw men off the scent.

Women are intrinsically secretive creatures and are even more secretive about their sexuality so when men start prying (which happens a lot) they will just deny that they ever think about sex and hope that the guy just goes away.

However if you know a girl really well, and she trusts what she tells you will go no further (a huge part of intimacy) and if you can loosen her up with a bit of

wine then you will be amazed
at what you hear.

You see the female mind is
much more complicated than
ours. It can process several
different thoughts and
emotions simultaneously and
is also much more sensitive to
emotive language than ours.

Women love to hear "dirty
talk" as long as it is real.
According to my expert panel,
you can't fake something like
that. It either comes from the
heart or not at all.

So if you are harboring these little things in your head when things really start getting heated between you and your girl, then let it fly and see how pleasantly shocked and aroused she will become.

One girl told me that she normally has lots of trouble reaching climax but one time with a particular "favorite" of hers, when things got really intense, he let out with:

*"You just love getting F*cked don't you, you dirty little thing".*

She said that hearing this from the man who turned her on so much when he was thrusting hard inside her absolutely blew her mind and threw her into the most intensive internal orgasms she has ever had.

So take it from the panel, open your mouth and start being comfortable engaging in dirty talk with your special girl.

Just let your natural sex drive
guide you on this one and it
will tell you what to do and
how far to go.

And don't overthink it. Just do
it and see how she reacts —
you will be pleasantly
surprised.

Dark Secret Number 2: Sensuality, Mood and "Connection"

Sensuality, Mood and "Connection" are essential - Before, during, and after, sex.

If you watch the average porn movie, what you normally see is a man undoing his clothes, getting a head job followed by sexual intercourse.

Whilst this might make sense
for a pornographic movie, it is
NOT how most women are in
reality.

The truth is, mostly all women
love sensuality, "romance"
and feeling an emotional
connection with the man
BEFORE and during sex, first.

First let's talk about
Sensuality, Romance and
Connection.

Well, we know that for guys,
they can just see a hot girl,

get a hard on and then a moment later, be ready to jump in the bedroom with her.

For women, it's much different.

Especially when a girl hasn't been dating a guy for a very long time, she usually needs more of a "revving up and warming up" period.

Guys think "foreplay" is just all the lesser sexual acts that you do once you've already hit the bedroom and you're leading up to the actual sex.

This isn't true. "Foreplay" for girls, is ALL the interactions with the guy, starting with the moment you first start hanging out, BEFORE and outside you even get to the bedroom.

It starts with you flirting with her a lot throughout the evening… teasing her… having fun with her… making her laugh.

Telling her she looks amazing.
Making her feel good and
having great conversations
with her that create a deeper
emotional connection with her.

Making great eye contact with
her, touching her and
caressing her throughout your
time together…teasing her.

Building up anticipation,
sexual tension and sexual
energy…

Giving her some soft, sensual kisses… and then a highly charged make out session.

Now, there are 2 types of "Sexual Energy" that you want to alternate between when you're with a girl.

THIS is what all women deeply CRAVE from all men… and what gets them REALLY going.

The 1st Is slower, "Sensual/ Romantic Energy."

Think of this kind of energy
like slower, more sensual,
softer kissing and making out,
caressing her, telling her she
looks gorgeous and bringing
her close to you…

Think of it like "making love".
It's more tender and romantic
and sensual.

Women need this kind of
energy and sensuality from
you, especially in the
beginning when they haven't
slept with you yet.

They need this so that they feel comfortable with you, they feel they can trust you and you aren't just treating them like a sex object or whore.

The 2nd sexual energy is "Aggressive Sexual Energy"

THIS kind of energy, is what "fucking" is. When you're in this kind of sexual energy, you are being more primal with her, more aggressive, more "predator" like.

Some examples of this would be: You are kissing her softly while you're having drinks at the bar…

Or you placing your hand on the back of her neck softly playing with her hair…

Then you suddenly **biting her bottom lip**, you pull her hair a bit and you say *"Mmmmm. I want you so bad right now."*

Or you're walking with her then you suddenly grab her,

and throw her against a wall
or car *(without banging up her
head though)* and giving her a
passionate, aggressive kiss.

It's whispering in her ear dirty
things, like:

*"You look so fucking hot right
now, I cannot WAIT to have
you"*

*"You just wait. You're not
going to be able to walk in the
morning."*

You switch into this
Aggressive Mode when
you've already been having
some slower sensual sex with
her.

You grab her and throw her on
top of the countertop, bite her
neck, grab the back of her
head and pull her hair,
squeeze her neck start
fucking her **hard.**

You get the idea? But you
want to alternate between
those 2 modes: **Sensual and
Aggressive.** You can

alternate between those 2 even several times during a sex session.

Women LOVE that contrast.

Get good at passionate KISSING

My panel told me that whilst caressing, oral sex and manual stimulation are very important during sex if they are not preceded by some good, passionate kissing then they can seem almost mechanical and without feeling.

So the advice of my panel is to become a great kisser and be great at making out — yeah sounds simple…

But some men aren't that great at kissing, only when you've kissed with passion and you got her all hot and heavy then you can proceed into all the raunchy stuff.

The other factor many men fail to consider is mood and

lighting. Women are very sensitive to these things and if they are not taken care of then no matter what you do to her, and how well you do it, she will always be a little turned off making it harder for her to enjoy herself and reach climax.

Now fellas, you don't have to go overboard and lay flowers on the bed and cover her in rose water but you do have to make some effort.

That means you have low
lighting, clean sheets, and a
clean room (no dirty socks on
the floor), nice smells and
nice music if you can manage
it.

This may sound like a lot but
all it really means is:

- Keep your room and
  house CLEAN
- Turn down the light -
  Bright lights are NOT
  sexy (women are self
  conscious when naked
  so dim the lights)

- Turn on some nice music but nothing too cheesy though
- Light a candle or two that smells nice.

When it's broken down in point form like the above, it's not that hard is it?

For this small amount of effort on your behalf, your woman will climax so much more easily and start to fall in love with a man who knows how to look after himself — and

seems to genuinely care
about her.

Ask any magician or hypnotist
and they will tell you that if
you are trying to influence
someone's mind and affect
their thoughts, then you
cannot have any distracting
features around.

This is why a hypnotist will
always be clean shaven, well
dressed and smell good. This
is so you focus on their words
and thoughts and not on their

disheveled appearance or
poor hygiene.

People trust people who look
good and take care of
themselves, so take a leaf out
of their book and do the same
because making a woman fall
in love with you is just another
form of hypnosis whether they
(or you) know it or not.

Now, if you have done all this
correctly then you should start
to feel your girl enjoying
herself and rubbing her body
against yours.

At this point start by lightly touching her breasts, just lightly at first but then gently squeezing more firmly later on which leads us into the 3rd secret...

Dark Secret Number 3: Mix It Up a Bit

Women love novelty and soon get bored with the same old kiss, rub and fondle, penetrate regime.

Be confident to involve toys into your sex play and always make it fun — just don't try to be too serious.

The more light hearted things are, the more women tend to

let go, and having intense orgasms is all about letting go.

Always aim to make sex fun, playful and passionate — just don't try to be too serious or "mechanical". A lot of guys focus on "performing" but that just makes it odd for her because she knows you're trying too hard.

Women care much more about a man who seems to be really present with her, connected with her, and

passionate in the moment
with her rather than focused
on his "performance".

The more present you are
with her, and passionate your
energy is, the more she will
LOVE it and it will feel that
much more intense for her.

The other 2 things you should
remember to do while leading
up to sex, and during the sex,
that will make her feel even
more relaxed with you and
unlock sexual desires are:

TALK TO HER: Be vocal and verbal all throughout. Positive affirmations and telling her numerous times:

How amazing her body is…

How HOT she is…

Say her tits are freakin' gorgeous…

Tell her she tastes sooo good when you're going downtown….

When you finally penetrate inside her, tell her a few times how tight she is, and tell her oh my God she feels sooo good. Moan throughout…

Don't be silent. Silence is not sexy for ANYONE, and women LOVE it when her man is groaning (in a masculine voice), say "Mmmm" and getting really into it.

EYE CONTACT: Some guys make the horrible mistake of not making eye contact a lot

with their girl during sex or
looking away, closing their
eyes, or staring at her vagina
the whole time.

That's the biggest mistake,
because then she feels like
you're totally disconnected
and not present, she's not
going to be into it like you are.

She wants to feel you THERE
with her. So, stare at her
sometimes in her eyes, like
you're hungry for her.

Almost like you're in a trance, and you're hypnotizing her as well.

It might be awkward for some guys to do this, but that's why it takes major confidence to do this — and why women love it so much when some guys does this — it shows you are fearless, confident, and passionate.

Kiss her sometimes on her lips, her neck and her shoulders. But the more you make confident, hungry eye contact with her, the more intense she will feel and will usually cum super intensely.

You don't have to make eye contact with her the ENTIRE time, but, maybe 60-70%.

The more you keep things playful and passionate with her, the more women tend to RELAX and let go, and having intense orgasms is all about getting her as relaxed, comfortable and confident as possible.

This then allows her to really tap into her feminine side and allow her to totally let go.

Remember that girls love to fantasise so asks her about something that she thinks about a lot and try to involve that in your play.

It could be putting on a uniform, tying her down and pretending she is your prisoner.

Remember that as much as women will deny it, they love being dominated.

Many members of my panel admit that they love being either tied or held down and taken by force with a man they trust and know so that they can almost pretend they are being raped (hey, don't judge - I'm not a rapist).

This last admission from most of my panel had me quite shocked, but at the same time from an animalistic perspective it also makes perfect sense.

In the animal kingdom the strongest males are often the ones who have the most female partners and quite often they take them by force.

Again, don't confuse this by forcing sex on her when she wants to stop. This mean you always have a safe word just in case one of you wants time out and remember to keep it fun.

Dark Secret
Number 4: Breasts
for Success

Did you know that if properly stimulated the female breast can cause a woman to have an intense, toe curling orgasm?

Did you know that if you suck on your girlfriend's breasts in a particular way it will release a hormone called oxytocin into her blood stream?

Oxytocin as a hormone
makes her bond with you so
intensely that she will start to
feel as though you are an
extension of her own body.

According to the panel, many
of the best men they have
ever been with really know
how to play with boobs.

I don't just mean a grope or
tickle, I'm talking about using
them as a gateway into a
woman's sexual soul.

From all the techniques I heard from my experts, one stood out more than any others and all the girls raved about it.

Here's your guideline to Breasts for Success:

Start by placing your mouth completely over your girls nipple so that it covers the aureolas (the pink ring around the nipple) and even some of the surrounding skin.

Then start sucking the nipple and the surrounding skin up into your mouth. Just gently at first and when you feel the nipple in your mouth becoming firmer, relax the pressure and let the nipple fall back down towards the skin.

But when it gets there instead of sucking again, keep the seal around the nipple and blow gently to create a mild pressure on top of the breast.

Then proceed back to gently creating suction in your mouth

again so that the nipple once again rises into your mouth but his time use more force.

Hold the breast in your mouth under suction, flicking your tongue back and forwards over the nipple to make it go even harder and then once again relax the pressure and blow the breast down onto the chest again.

This sucking and blowing technique gradually builds up the intensity and makes most women go wild. It tickles them in a way that gets right down into their bones and turns on their sexual machinery like the flick of a switch.

One of the girls told me that this technique done correctly is guaranteed to get her dripping wet and ready for climax at the drop of a hat. Another told me that it is not the sort of thing that a girl forgets easily.

Dark Secret Number 5: Heading Downstairs

Okay boys, now that we have kissed and caressed its time to start touching her private parts. Remember that going here too early is a major turnoff and will only put pressure on her to get aroused.

So don't rush into this one and wait till she is moaning

and rubbing her groin against you before you even think about touching her "down there".

There are exceptions to this rule but for right now just trust the expert panel as they tell no lies. Why would they? They are not your girlfriend and therefore don't have to lie to stroke your precious ego.

According to the panel the best way to start warming her up down below is to **leave her pants on to start with.**

Just brush your hand against her skirt or jeans over where her private parts are with a gentle pressure and then move it away again. Tease her.

Girls love to be teased, it gives you value and is also very playful and when it comes to sexual liaisons — playful is always a good thing.

Once you have touched her a few times and your are ready to get a bit more adventurous,

start by unzipping or
unbuttoning her pants just a
little bit.

Touch her around the top of
her pubic line and run the tips
of your fingers up towards her
hip line.

This creates an electric thrill
effect that will give her goose
bumps and further sensitize
the area.

Next, unzip her even further
and now place your fingers
further down but not inside

her underwear. Not yet
anyway.

Just tickle around her clitoral
area and labia, gentle
touching this area through her
panties. When she can't stand
it anymore, start rubbing her
through her pants first around
the clitoral area but also
around the lower labia.

Feel for the hardening clitoris
though the pants. That should
be your focus but you can
also excite her by pushing
your fingers into the area

where her vaginal opening will
be.

You will only be able to push
in for maybe a centimeter or
two as her underwear will be
in the way but this will only
drive her even more crazy.

Because you will start to
touch her inner parts (which
are very sensitive), this will
make her want more but the
panties will stop you going
any further.

Hopefully by this stage you will start to feel her wetness coming though the pants. This means she is starting to get going and soon will be ready for more.

Your next move is to put your hands down her pants and start feeling her with your skin touching hers. If you have done everything right she will be warm and wet with a firm clitoris that will be as sensitive as the tip of your penis when it is erect.

Start by massaging her clitoris is a circular or side to side motion with your middle finger and use the index finger and fourth finger to massage the lips on either side of the clit.

This alone can give a girl an incredibly intense clitoral orgasms. Whilst you are doing this, remember to make sure though that you are holding and kissing her at the same time.

Remember to take care of her upstairs as well as her

downstairs. Kiss her neck and bite her ears gently. Combining two erogenous zones at the same time can be an incredible turn on.

Make sure to help her out of her panties at this stage so that you can start to put your fingers inside her.

Remember that even though girls do love deep penetration, one of the most sensitive parts of the vagina is the G spot which is located just inside on the upper wall.

It should feel a bit rough due to all the nerve endings and rubbing this area will make her go wild. See if you can stimulate her clitoris and penetrate her with your fingers at the same time.

She will love you for it and you will give her intense orgasms just from this alone.

Remember that many girls also like to feel your dick during foreplay as it turns them on to feel how hard you are.

So if she hasn't already, you can guide her hand to your dick as you are stimulating her to show her how much she turns you on.

To really get her going though we will have to proceed to a technique that the French call "le sexe oral". And that leads us into our secret…

Dark Secret Number 6: Tongues Are Not Just For Talking…

So here it comes guys. One of the most important things that I am going to tell you.

Most women love oral sex. It creates a sensation that is like no other that you can give a woman and whilst foreplay, kissing, caressing and stimulation by hand can feel great….

Using your mouth and tongue correctly on a woman's private parts will send her into a seventh heaven.

After you have played gently with your girls breasts and worked her up enough to take off her pants, lie her down on her back with her legs spread and start kissing her chest.

Then keep going down kissing her stomach, pelvis and inner thighs. Remember to tease her and build up the anticipation for what is coming. When you think she has suffered enough torment in waiting, heads towards the warm wet spot.

Start by just gently blowing on it. Blow then stop. Blow then stop. Now get you index and middle finger and part the top of the upper lips so that you expose the clitoris and clitoral hood.

Start by gently flicking it with the tip of your tongue, adding more and more pressure and you proceed. Once you have gotten into a rhythm, put your mouth over the clitoris and surrounding skin and suck it gently into your mouth creating a mild vacuum.

This will encourage blood flow into the clit and outer lips making this area much more sensitive. After this put your mouth over the clitoris and move your tongue over the clitoris from side to side.

Make sure you alter the speed intensity and rhythm as you

go as the same stimulus repeated too many times becomes boring.

Remember to lift your mouth off the skin every now and then as this will allow for a rush of cool air to come through and evaporate the wetness of the skin (she should be very moist by now indeed).

This alternating cool and hot sensation is one of the most pleasurable things about oral

sex and should be repeated
throughout the whole process.

After you have been doing
this for a while your girl should
be building closer and closer
towards orgasm. Don't be
afraid to start putting your
whole mouth over your girls
pussy. Suck on it like you
would the froth of the top of a
cappuccino.

Gently but with enough force
to be felt. Don't be intimidated
by the vagina, start
experimenting but always

make sure you are focussing on the clitoris most of the time.

If you feel like you need a break then poke your tongue out as far as you can and start thrusting it inside your girls pussy like a small penis. Lick inside and around the inner labia. Just go for it and your girl will never forget what you have done for her.

As you feel her hips starting to gyrate then focus again on the clitoris rubbing it backwards

and forwards with your
tongue.

Don't stop for more than a few
seconds at a time as she is
getting more and more
excited.

Remember that whilst you are
licking her clit you can also
slide your fingers inside her
and play with her G spot at
the same time.

If your girls hasn't come from
just oral sex then giving her
digital penetration at the same

time will definitely put her over the edge.

Let's look at one of the greatest womanizers of all time – Carlos the jackal.

Now Carlos was a clever fellow you see. He knew how to make them fall in love with him with a mix of kindness and harsh reprimands that made women feel like they were special and cared for while also in the presence of a strong masculine presence.

What was also reported about Carlos was that he was amazing in bed and was able to connect with women very deeply, and do things to a woman's body that would make her crave him even when he was not around.

One of the main things Carlos was renowned for was oral sex but he never put himself into a state of submission when he did it.

According to one of Carlos's many woman he was able to

control her body and make her climax on command.

No matter what he was doing he was always in control and put his girls into a trance like state of submission. He always had a "dangerous" and intense energy about him too when he was in his sexual hungry mode with a woman… Almost like he was in a trance.

"You never knew if he was going to kill you or fuck you"

This was what one of the woman reported, and it was exactly that mix of intimacy and darkness that gave him such an edge.

Dark Secret Number 7: A Time to Fuck...

Now as we have talked about already, women are complicated creatures. Unlike men who can "get it up" at the drop of a hat, woman need to be revved up and "warmed up" over time like starting an old car.

As we stated earlier, the "warming and revving up" time starts really the moment you first see her.

And then you keep building it up… building the sexual energy and tension… Flirting with her, teasing her, etc. throughout the day or evening.

You need to spend time on them making them feel comfortable and increasingly more aroused as they start to let themselves go bit by bit.

Once you have done this well, any woman will tell you that they start feeling the need to have something inside them

and the good news for us is
that is the part most of us
enjoy the most — penetration.

So once you have set the
mood, caressed and kissed
our woman followed up by
fondling and also potentially
oral sex then you should
reach a point where your girl
is so wet and sensitive that
the mere slip of a finger inside
her pussy sends them into
convulsions of pleasure.

It is at this point that your hard
dick comes into play and can
be used to its full extent.

So after talking to the panel about the sexual positions they found to be most pleasurable - I found that there were a few that stood out far above the rest and there was also one gem that not everybody knew about.

After much debating with my angels I managed to nail it down to the top 5 positions available. Now I can give you 10 but in all honesty, you just need a handful that you can remember.

5 orgasmic sex positions
that are guaranteed to make
her scream, come so hard
that she will come back for
more.

What is important to
remember as well with
penetration is that variety is
important in in speed and
intensity.

It's also important to vary
between the 2 different types
of sexual energy: Sensual/
Romantic Sexual Energy
(usually better to start with,
especially the first few times

you have sex with a new girl),
and then Aggressive Sexual
Energy.

If she is really enjoying herself
in one certain position though,
then stick to what you are
doing and gradually build up
the intensity.

If you feel that she is not that
into it then slow down and
change to a new position,
kissing her nipples, lips and
neck during the change to
keep her aroused.

So without further ado…

CHAPTER TWO
Orgasmic Sex Positions

Orgasmic Sex Position 1. Missionary Position

This tried and tested position can be fun but is normally just a great way to start things off.

Start by gently rubbing the nob of your penis around the outside of her lips and even against her clitoris.

This will give her a great thrill and should also get your

penis wet as she should be dripping by now.

After teasing your girl for a minute or so then push just the end of your penis into and out of her vagina but not so deep just at this moment.

Remember some girls need to get used to having something inside them so shoving your penis in all at once can be quite painful if you do it too quickly.

Women LOVE the "build-up."
Women LOVE anticipation.
So, draw it out. Tease it out.
Don't put it all in at once…

A little bit at a time. Think of it
like you're torturing her… You
don't let her have all at once.
She'll love being teased and
tortured like that.

Remember too that most of
the nerve endings inside the
vagina are in the first 2-3cm
so just putting your end in can
also be very pleasurable in

itself even without full penetration.

Now you can start pushing further in, a little bit more with every thrust, until you get to a point where you are more than half way then you should push all the way in using one thrust.

This major movement all the way into the back of your girl's vagina is a great thrill for women as when deep penetration occurs the cervix is stimulated which can be very pleasurable.

Now that you are fully inside your girl, take advantage of her.

Girls like to be dominated a little bit so get right on top of her and let her feel your full weight. Grab both her ass cheeks in your hand and squeeze them hard sometimes as you go inside her.

Try to create more of a gliding motion as you fuck and not to do too much "pounding," as girls typically don't like that super fast "pounding like a jackhammer" movement, unlike what pornos may have you believe.

The very back is where her G spot is and it is very sensitive to rubbing during penetration.

If you can manage it, arch your back and use one hand to support yourself and whilst you fuck your girl use your other hand (normally your right) to rub her clitoris externally.

Not all girls bodies are shaped right for this but if you can pull this one off, it can be magic.

Orgasmic Sex Position 2: Into The Lotus

From the missionary, the next position to easily get into is where you put your girls legs back behind her with your arms and enter her from on top giving a very deep penetration into the vagina.

Try to angle the hips here as well so as to get full stimulation of the G spot. Start by going slowly and then speed up as your girl gets excited.

As both of your arms are used up here try to see if your girl would like to play with herself at the same time.

NOTE: NOT ALL girls like this position, however. For some girls, I've found that especially some more smaller and petite girls, they can find this position uncomfortable or even painful.

So, as usual and with ALL positions and moves you put

on a girl, you can get your
answer easily and rather
quickly if you just tune into
her, listen and observe.

*Did she suddenly stop
moaning as much?*

*Did she get quiet altogether?
Is she not smiling or does her
face look like it's wincing or
uncomfortable?*

If so, you may want to only
stay in that position a minute
or two and then try bringing
her legs down a bit more

closer to the missionary position.

Some girls are just not that flexible, either!

Rotate your girl around to different angles when you fuck her from this position and see what she responds to best.

When you find that position that she moans the loudest in and responds to the best, really start to go for it and watch your girls eyes get wider and she screams for more.

Remember to be comfortable
sometimes alternating
between "slower, sensual
energy" and "aggressive
sexual energy," and
dominating your girl during
sex at times.

*Don't ask for permission just
do it.*

Orgasmic Sex Position 3: Gangnam Style

This position was coined Gangnam style by one of the girls because the first time her lover did this to her the song gangnam style was playing in the background.

It's difficult to describe this position in words but when you get it you will know.

Basically you lean over your
girl pushing her legs right
back so that her knees are
essentially touching her
elbows.

Your hands are placed at this
point next to her shoulders on
either side and the inside of
your forearm is pushing her
legs back.

Then take your hands and put
them round the back of her
shoulders so that your fingers
are coming up over the top of
her back.

In this position her legs are pinned back and your bodies are very close due to the fact that you are holding her essentially by the top of her back with your hands on the top of her shoulders coming from behind her with your finger facing your body.

In this position what you are now able to do is very rapidly and firmly fuck your girl by pulling her back into you whilst you thrust into her at the same time.

You get very deep penetration and maximum stimulation of her G spot, at the same time as her hips are angled back towards her head as well.

If you can get this right and start thrusting very quickly and firmly you can also get your pelvis rubbing against her clitoris for added affect.

I have used this position a few times myself already and have given two girls the first "internal" orgasm they have ever had.

What amazes me most about this position is how quickly they achieved this orgasms as well.

One of these girls only took about 30 seconds each time prompting her to say to me that it was "too easy" for me to get her off and it "wasn't fair for the other guys".

Please note as well though that not all body shapes are

able to perform this position
and normally it works best
when the guy is taller and the
girl is shorter.

But again, some girls may be
uncomfortable or painful in
this position.

So as with all positions, tune
in to your girl, listen to her,
look at her, and see how she's
responding. If she has quieted
the moans, it might not be a
good position for her.

Orgasmic Sex Position 4: In the Dog

So here we are at every guys favourite position and if you believe the porn stars and the 1800 numbers, every girls favourite position as well.

Whilst it would be logical to think that in fact everything we hear from porn stars and dodgy porn sites is just set up to take out money, the reality is that many women love

doggy style just as much as
men do and for good reason.

Doggy style is the epitome of
male dominated sex and as
we have already discussed
women love to be dominated
in bed (and out of it) even
though they might not want to
admit it.

Doggy style also give great
deep penetration and also
gives you the ability to reach
around and play with her clit
at the same time you are
inside her.

If you just want to concentrate on penetration then get your girl to play with herself to give both internal and clitoral stimulation.

Doggy style also allows you to play it up a bit as it is an animalistic position that really can bring out the beast in both of you.

Try pulling back on her hair lightly as you are thrusting into her from behind. If she really likes this then pull a little harder so that her neck is strained backwards.

This creates a feeling of restriction like being tied down to the bed and again its about domination and power and yes most women love it.

Remember when you are in this position to play with her ass cheeks. Get them in your hands and squeeze them firmly.

Rub them around with your hands and if she is getting

into it give her a light smack on the ass. If she likes this then you can do this a little harder.

Not too many times though or it will wear thin. Most women like a little bit of pleasure spiked with pain but just don't overdo it. Learn to read your woman's body and know when she is peaking.

 If you are feeling a bit cheeky and if you think your girl can handle it then get your little

finger and place gentle
pressure on your girls bum.

Just outside at first, and then
if she seems okay with it
gently move it inside her ass
just enough to complement
what you are dong from
behind already.

Its true that not all girls like
anal sex but mostly all girls if
they feel comfortable with you
will allow you to just gently
play with their bottom during
sex.

If you find that she really likes
this stimulation then you
never know, maybe in the
future she will let you put your
member inside her back door.

Orgasmic Sex Position 5: Spooning

According to my panel of sexperts, one very underrated position in the sexual repertoire of most men is the spoon.

Spooning has been around since the dawn of time and has been very popular and for very good reason.

Spooning allows for the man to take control of his woman from behind whilst getting a great deep penetration angle that also stimulates the G spot as well.

Add to this the fact that you can also put your hand around the front and give your girl a nice clitoral massage at the same time and whammo we have an instant winner.

As you are at the back of your girl's head during this you can also get her to turn her head

toward yours and give her
very sensual kisses at the
same time all this is going on.

If she just wants to rest her
head forwards and enjoy what
you are doing to her then you
can gently kiss her neck and
nibble on her ear and her
neck which is also a great turn
on.

Many couples love this
position especially in the
morning as you don't have to
breath morning breath all over
each other and for those who

like a bit of anal sex every
now and then then spooning
position also offers a great
way to go there as well.

So to make sure that you are
giving your girl the best she
can get, make sure to use the
spoon on her.

So there you have it, a
manual on how to get your girl
off!

Remember this is not from my
own mind, this is from the girls
who know best and who were

willing to share their secrets with us.

Get Harder & Last Longer Naturally

I don't know about you but as a guy, I'm always on the lookout for methods that makes me harder and last longer in bed without any major side effects.

Hacks to improve sexual performance, stamina and more importantly, salvage hurt egos.

There's been some exercises and herbs that have been

proven effective in delaying ejaculation. Here are 7 tips that work:

Tip 1: Kegel Exercises

Perhaps the most popular exercise to improve men's performance in bed is the Kegel exercise. It involves the pubococcygeal or PC muscles which control semen and urine flow.

When controlled, the PC muscles can boost the firmness of the penis and

even boost ejaculation.
What's great with this exercise
is that it can be done
anywhere, anytime without
anyone knowing it.

Kegel exercise results to
better sex since men can
delay their ejaculation, control
their orgasm and boost the
size of their penis.

The best way to determine
where the PC muscles are
would be to stop the flow of
urine. Once you have
familiarize yourself where
your PC muscles are, you can

start performing the Kegel exercise.

It's very simple, just tighten the PC muscles and release it repeatedly for five-seconds. You can then increase the time you hold on to the PC muscles as you progress.

Tip 2: Stop And Squeeze During Sex

The stop and squeeze method is a simple method done during sex, just before you're about to explode.

When you're close to coming, stop and squeeze the head of your penis using your thumb and forefinger and apply pressure on the urethra.

The urethra is the tube which runs along the underside of your penis. It temporarily decreases sexual tension by pushing blood out of the penis, and allows you to last longer in bed.

Tip 3: Take Kava Root

You would be surprised to know that the foods you eat

can influence your performance in bed. Certain natural herbs can prolong sex with minimal side effects.

One of these herbs for longer lasting sex is the kava root. It increases the flow of blood to the penis and decreases the reaction to increased sexual stimuli.

By taking 100 milligrams of kava before sexual intercourse, you can enjoy longer lasting sex.

Tip 4: Hibiscus Flower Essence

Hibiscus flower essence can also make you last longer in bed. It relieves stress and enhances the ability to sustain an erection. Two drops of hibiscus flower essence is mixed with ¼ cup of water which you can take daily.

Tip 5: Gingko Biloba

Ginkgo Biloba has been around for centuries and have been used by the ancient Chinese for medicinal purposes. In a study by the University of Maryland Medical Center, it has been proven effective in increasing the libido in men.s

Ginkgo biloba works by opening up blood vessels, increasing blood flow to the penis and improving circulation. It's considered as anti-depressant for sexual dysfunction.

The standard recommended dosage of ginkgo biloba is 40-80mg, 3 times a day (up to 240mg/day).

Tip 6: Tongkat Ali

Tongkat Ali is a flowering plant that grows in Southeast Asia and literally means "Ali's Walking Stick" in reference to its ability to enhance sexual performance in men.

It's a natural treatment to premature ejaculation, improves libido and increases testosterone levels in men. In various laboratory animal tests, the herb has been proven to increase the sexual activity of mature rats.

Various Tongkat Ali supplements are sold in the market. According to the late Dr. Azizol Abdul Kadir of Malaysia who made extensive research on the herb, the recommended daily dosage of Tongkat Ali is 200mg.

Tip 7: Yohimbe

Yohimbe comes from the bark of the West African evergreen and is also very popular in Chinese medicine.

It is used for sexual dysfunction and acts as a

powerful aphrodisiac, thereby improving sexual desire. It too increases blood flow to the genitals of both men and women.

I find that taking Yohimbine 5 mgs at 30-60 mins prior to sexual activity always works for me.

Keep Her Coming Back For More

The secret in getting her coming back for more? DO EXACTLY as outlined in this book. Go back and read this book again until you can memorize the moves.

However let's sum up the highlights:

- Girls are just as **dirty** as we are and the trick is bringing it out of them

- Be confident with your woman and take control and don't take sex too seriously, it's there to be enjoyed and its great for you on so many levels to learn how to let go and just enjoy the moment.

- Try different things and don't be afraid to just let go and enjoy yourself. Sex can be a lot of fun if you are willing to try different things and women love a guy who is confident enough to experiment with them.

- Make sure to set the
mood and never under-
estimate the power of a
sexual sensual kiss to
get things going.
- Learn to enjoy foreplay
and getting your girl wet
and ready before
jumping into the
penetration part of sex.
Getting your girl off and
enjoying yourself should
go hand in hand.
- Become a master of oral
sex and you will never
be short of fuck buddies

- When it does come time
to go inside your partner,
learn to take it easy and
vary the intensity rhythm
and position to get the
most out of your sexual
experience.
- MASTER the 5
Orgasmic sex positions
and follow them to a tee.
These 5 positions have
worked on women of all
shapes, sizes and races.
- And above all have fun
and don't worry too
much if things don't

always work out.
Seriously.

The great thing about sex is
that you can always do it
again, and again, and again…

That's a wrap, now go and
have a good fuckin time!

Alex X

Free Gift

Download "10 Tools For Stronger Erections" At: http://bit.ly/10strongerection

So you know how to make her come using orgasmic sex positions but do you want to get stronger erections?

Download this check list and get the 10 tools to help you with stronger erections so that you can last longer in bed.

Download "10 Tools For Stronger Erections" At: http://bit.ly/10strongerection

Thank You... And One Tiny Favor, Please

Thank you for reading my book! I really value your feedback and would appreciate it if you could leave a review.

As an independent author, I have a heart for helping people by sharing the information presented in this book.

Please leave me a helpful
review on Amazon right now
by turning to the last page.

It would really help benefit
other people and Zeus my
doggy values your opinion as
well!

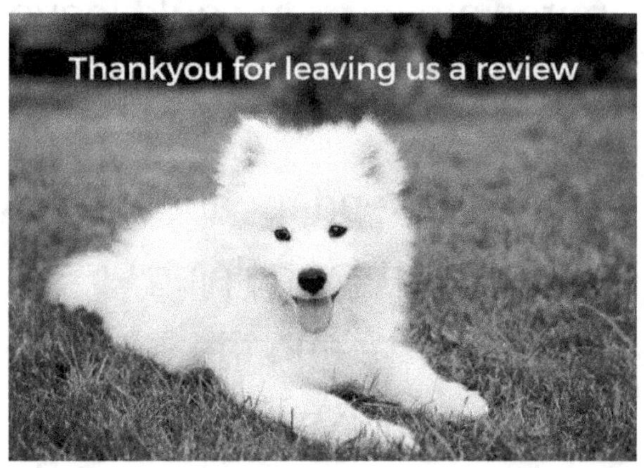